APPLE CIDER VINEGAR

The most comprehensive step-by-step guide
for total health and weight loss

KIRSTEN YANG

TABLE OF CONTENT

INTRODUCTION

Apple Cider Vinegar (ACV) is made by crushing fresh, organically grown apples and allowing them to mature in wooden barrels. This boosts natural fermentation and allows the vinegar to mature.

It is an effective natural bacteria-fighting agent that contains many vital minerals and trace elements such as potassium, calcium, magnesium, phosphorous, chlorine, sodium, sulfur, copper, iron, silicon and fluorine that are vital for a healthy body.

There are so many people in the world nowadays who are so conscious of their weight and figure. It is due to the influence of media which is emphasizing on the standard weight of a person.

Fashion is also considered as a factor because they mostly cater to those who are size 0 than to those people who were born to become size 12. There have been many people who became interested in weight loss and made good and bad information about it.

There are only a few of useful information but still so many are not helpful or just a bogus. If you really want to lose weight rapidly then I believe the best diet for you is apple cider vinegar diet?

If you are just living very far from civilization and not having your own television then you might not know or have heard about the diet which is about at the top of the list of natural remedies on the history of mankind.

This diet according to research was seen in Egypt about 3000 BC and in China about 1200 BC. Back in that time, the apple cider vinegar is considered to be used as a reagent for pickling and also used as food.

These apples are needed to be processed in order to become a cider vinegar. Apples that are used must be fresh and not undergone any pasteurization in order to become a cider vinegar.

In order to accumulate acids and enzymes, they are not just using fresh apples but also vinegars to help in the fermentation process.

Apple cider vinegar diet will not just help the person to lose weight but also it is a good way in increasing magnesium, fiber, and pectin within our body that is water soluble.

CHAPTER 1

WHAT IS APPLE CIDER VINEGAR?

Apple cider vinegar has been known as an effective anti-bacterial substance for a long time. It contains a number of nutrients which are known to be good for skin, and overall good health.

These include Calcium, Iron, fluorine, magnesium, and potassium. In its natural form, Apple cider vinegar is made taking organically grown apples and crushing them, collecting the juices into wooden barrels.

The apple juice's fermentation is enhanced by the use of a natural (untreated) wooden barrel and matures to develop cloudy dark bacterial foam referred to as mother.

This mother foam adds a variety of enzymes and minerals to the apple cider vinegar that is not present with more mainstream (high production) fermentation processes. Additionally, the mother from one batch can be re-used in future batches to speed and assist the brewing process.

Apple cider vinegar cures a lot of ills. Ailments such as arthritis, constipation, acne, gout, sore throats, high blood pressure, weight issues and a myriad of other health issues can be helped and even cured by drinking apple cider vinegar.

What makes it so special that it can be used as a remedy for these health problems and why is it better than other vinegar? It's the nutritional value that's in apple cider vinegar that makes it a powerhouse against various illnesses.

This vinegar is made from freshly crushed apples that are put in wooden barrels to allow for natural fermentation. Natural cider vinegar should be a rich brown color. When you look at it in the light you will see brownish particles that resemble cobwebs. This substance is called the "mother". As it ages you will see more of the mother accumulate in the bottom of the bottle.

Natural apple cider vinegar has a pungent odor which is a good sign. There's an abundance of healthy nutrients in the "mother substance". Unfiltered natural organic apple cider vinegar has proven powerful health benefits.

Some of the nutrients that give it its healing powers are iron, copper, trace elements, phosphorous, silicon, essential amino acids, sulphur, magnesium, natural organic sodium, natural organic fluorine, and many other powerful nutrients.

One nutrient that Apple cider vinegar is loaded with that holds the key to youthfulness is potassium. Potassium helps build and maintain youthful and healthy tissues.

Potassium also helps to slow down the hardening and clogging process that can murder the cardiovascular system.

The vinegar you see on supermarket shelves are all devoid of nutritional value because this vinegar are distilled and pasteurized which means that the "mother" has been removed.

Most people use vinegar as a flavoring and aren't thinking of it as a nutritional drink. Vinegar producers aren't in the business of educating the public on the powerful health benefits of natural apple cider vinegar because they aren't aware of these benefits.

It's really sad because people are missing out on the great flavor that it adds to foods along with the nutritional value it has for a product that has no nutritional value and can cause more harm than good.

The regular vinegar you see on store shelves is distilled, pasteurized vinegar, which people prefer only because they aren't aware of what they are actually consuming. If they were educated about apple cider vinegar, they would choose it over the commercial vinegar.

People tend to think that the clear vinegar is healthy because it looks clean but it only looks like that because it has been stripped of all its nutritional value. Consuming this vinegar can be bad for your health.

Commercial vinegar does not have any vitamins, minerals or potassium that the body needs.

Don't let the way it looks deter you from using it. The brownish color with sediment at the bottom of the bottle doesn't look as good as the crystal clear vinegar you see in the supermarket.

The proof is not in how it looks but how it can change your health. With all the great benefits that it has to offer it only makes sense to incorporate it into your daily health regimen.

What doesn't hurt you can only make you stronger and has proven that it can strengthen your health by providing you with the much-needed nutrients your body needs.

HISTORY OF APPLE CIDER VINEGAR

Apple cider vinegar is perhaps the number one natural remedy chronicled throughout human history. The use of vinegar as a tonic has been documented as far back as 5000 BC by the Babylonians who were using the date palm to make wine and vinegar. They used it as a food and as a pickling agent.

Vinegar residues have been found in ancient Egyptian urns dated 3000 BC. Chinese historical documents from 1200 BC tout the glories of vinegar benefits as well.

The reasons for its popular medicinal use and as an energizing drink are scientifically well-founded by modern science also. Apple cider vinegar benefits are a result of its source - the noble apple - famous for the saying an apple a day keeps the doctor away.

Apples contain not only vitamins, minerals, and antioxidants, but also dietary fiber. In addition, they contain virtually no fat or sodium.

All of the apple goodness is miraculously transferred to apple cider vinegar especially when it's left unprocessed. Apple cider vinegar made from whole apples and not pasteurized or filtered contains not only all of the apple's nutrients but also many additional enzymes and organic acids produced during the two fermentations required to turn apples into vinegar.

Braggs Apple Cider Vinegar is the most popular brand that meets all of the requirements needed to reap the treasured benefits of ACV.

The long list of apple cider benefits ranges from an antiseptic to an antioxidant while providing a host of absorbable minerals such as potassium and magnesium including pectin, and a water-soluble fiber, which is one of the many reasons for the success of the cider vinegar diet.

The recommended method of using apple cider vinegar is to make it into a tonic by mixing 2 or 3 teaspoons of apple cider vinegar in an 8-ounce glass of water and drinking it before or during each meal. One point to remember when taking apple cider vinegar between meals or before going to bed is to always rinse your mouth to avoid any prolonged vinegar contact with the enamel on your teeth.

As far as apple cider vinegar remedies are concerned the list literally ranges from A to Z. It starts at acne and asthma and runs to warts and weight loss ending with yeast infections including such ailments as cancer, eczema, fatigue, fungus, headaches, heartburn, insomnia, sore throat, ulcers, and varicose veins in between - to list just a few.

In short, apple cider vinegar lives up to its reputation of being the simplest answer to perfect health and a timeless cure all as well.

A prize in any person's natural remedy medicine chest and a powerful preventative to whatever ails ya, not to forget its age old popularity as a world-class tonic. Make sure you always use pure unprocessed organic apple cider vinegar with the mother still in it, and you can rely on its amazing properties to help provide you and your family with a long and healthy life.

RAW APPLE CIDER VINEGAR A SUPER FOOD

It has been around for centuries and was used in both cooking and medicine. Manufactured from fermented whole apples, the best apple cider vinegar is raw.

That is to say, it has not been pasteurized, distilled or filtered as these processes can reduce the healthful properties of the vinegar.

Raw apple cider vinegar is best purchased from health food stores rather than grocery stores. This is because the vinegar sold for cooking is of a lower quality than the vinegar made for consumption as a health supplement.

When it comes to apple cider vinegar, it pays to read the label and get the best product you can find.

AN AGE-OLD REMEDY

For centuries, apple cider vinegar has been used as a medicinal remedy for a wide number of illnesses. At one time or another, it has been used as a treatment for warts, fighting infection, as an antiseptic and even to increase fertility!

While it's hard to say if this super food really helped any of these conditions, there is no doubt that it can be very useful for improving general health and helping with weight loss.

APPLE CIDER VINEGAR AND HEALTH

It's very rich in essential nutrients. Nutrients are vital for health. Without nutrients, such as vitamins and minerals, your cells, organs and bodily systems will not function properly and ill health is likely to follow.

Modern diets are often very low in essential nutrients and many people eat too much-processed food.

Processed food, as the term suggests, has been through a refining process to change the taste, texture and/or shelf life of the food and this usually means fewer or no healthful nutrients.

Many people's diets are very high in calories but low in essential nutrients so even an overweight and clearly overfed person can be suffering from malnutrition!

Consuming raw apple cider vinegar is an easy and convenient way to get a daily dose of essential nutrients.

So, what nutrients does this powerful food contain? It's quite a long list but apple cider vinegar (and remember, go for the raw stuff and avoid any vinegar that have been filtered, pasteurized or distilled) contains these and many other essential nutrients...

- Vitamin A

- Vitamin C

- Vitamin E

- Vitamin B1, B2, and B6

- Beta carotene (a form of vitamin A)

- Vitamin K

- Potassium

- Calcium

- Magnesium

- Phosphorous

- Copper

- Iron

There aren't many foods, raw or otherwise, that can boast such a wide variety of nutrients!

A POWER WEIGHT LOSS AID?

In addition to being a miraculous health food, apple cider vinegar has been shown to be very useful for fat loss.

With such a large proportion of the population overweight, many people are looking for ways to make the fat loss less of an ordeal.

Exercise, strict diets, certain drugs, and even surgery are all used in an effort to lose fat but recent research and plenty of anecdotal evidence suggest that good old raw apple cider vinegar can really help your fat loss efforts.

In numerous studies, apple cider vinegar has been shown to...

- Increase metabolism - the rate at which you burn calories

- Decreased appetite

- Increase energy and vitality

- Lower blood glucose levels

- Improve fat burning

In a 2004 study published by Science News Online, subjects reported a one pound per month fat loss while using apple cider vinegar despite not making any dietary or exercise changes!

Just imagine how much more effective apple cider vinegar would be if combined with some moderate dietary changes and regular exercise!

HOW TO USE APPLE CIDER VINEGAR?

If health is your aim, you should consume one tablespoon of apple cider vinegar first thing in the morning and the last thing at night.

This will ensure you get a good nutritional start to your day and also provide essential nutrients for the repair process that happens while you sleep.

If you are more interested in weight loss and as this food is an effective appetite suppressant, consume one tablespoon 15 minutes before all main meals. For most of us, this means one tablespoon three times a day.

If you are feeling hungry between meals, you could also try a tablespoon to ward off an unruly appetite.

As well as preventing hunger, this also means you get an extra shot of healthy vitamins and minerals.

IS IT SAFE FOR EVERYONE?

Apple cider vinegar is a 100% natural product and as such is safe for a vast majority of the population to use. Not only is it safe, if can help treat a huge number of medical conditions including:

- Arthritis

- High blood pressure

- Circulatory problems

- Depression

- Indigestion

- Digestive upsets

- Headaches

- Nasal congestion

- Rashes

- Ulcers

That being said, you should never attempt to self-medicate with apple cider vinegar and should always discuss your medical requirements with your family physician.

It's unlikely your doctor will tell you not to take this food but it's always better to be safe than sorry.

Providing your doctor gives the all clear, you might find that your condition and symptoms improve rapidly soon after you start taking apple cider vinegar.

Grab your spoon...!

It's clear that this super food is both healthy and useful for fat loss but only if you actually move from reading to doing. Make sure you get "apple cider vinegar with the mother."

It's relatively cheap, easy to get hold off and could be one of the best things you do for your health!

Now that you understand how Apple cider vinegar is a powerful weight loss aid.

CHAPTER 2

HOW TO MAKE RAW APPLE CIDER VINEGAR?

INGREDIENTS

- 3 small apples (core and peel included, no stem)

- 3 tsp raw sugar

- Filtered water to cover

INSTRUCTIONS

1.	Wash and chop your apples into medium sized pieces (or use the peels and cores of 6-7 small apples after making a pie). Place them in a clean, rinsed and sterilized wide mouth jar.

2.	Mix the sugar with 1 cup of water and pour on top of the apples.

3.	Add more water if needed to cover the apples.

4.	Cover the jar with a paper towel or cheesecloth and secure it with a band. This keeps nastiest away while letting the liquid breathe.

5. Place the jar in a warm, dark place for 2-3 weeks – I just kept it in my pantry.

6. Strain out the liquid and discard the apple pieces.

7. Return the liquid to the same jar and cover it again (same paper or cheesecloth).

8. Return the jar to the same warm, dark place and leave it to do its thing for roughly 4 to 6 weeks, stirring with a plastic or wooden spoon every few days or so.

9. After the first 4 weeks, you can begin to also taste your vinegar and once it reaches an acidity you like, you can actually transfer it to a bottle with a lid and begin using it.

Prep time: 5 mins

Total time: 2-3 months

CHAPTER 3

BENEFITS OF APPLE CIDER VINEGAR

Apple cider vinegar has been called a cure for everything. Health enthusiasts have used it for everything from acne and allergies to sore throats and warts. Vinegar in its many forms has been used for centuries for all sorts of folk remedies.

Recently with the flood of people turning to home and natural based remedies, apple cider vinegar has come to light as an especially useful health tonic.

People are often skeptical about something as common as apple cider vinegar is such an effective treatment for so many ailments. Folk remedy experts have long used it as a natural cure-all. Research conducted on the proposed benefits of apple cider vinegar have actually proven many claims correct.

Apple cider vinegar has a lot of benefits for your health. There are also many books written about apple cider vinegar describing how excellent it is for your health.

Proponents believe that Apple cider vinegar can cure or help with a myriad of diseases and health problems such as arthritis, osteoporosis, high blood pressure, high cholesterol, cancer, infection, indigestion, memory, and aging.

Also, the most talked-about benefit of apple cider vinegar apparently is its help with weight loss.

Here are some of the major benefits of Apple Cider Vinegar:

1. Apple Cider Vinegar And weight loss

2. Apple Cider Vinegar And Acid Reflux

3. Apple Cider Vinegar And Acne

4. Apple Cider Vinegar And Wart

5. Apple Cider Vinegar And Heartburn

6. Apple Cider Vinegar And Yeast Infection

7. Apple Cider Vinegar And Arthritis

8. Apple Cider Vinegar For Skin

9. Apple Cider Vinegar And Cholesterol

10. Apple Cider Vinegar For Hair

11. Apple Cider Vinegar And Blood Pressure

12. Apple Cider Vinegar For Sinus Infection

13. Apple Cider Vinegar And Candida

14. Apple Cider Vinegar And Gout

15. Apple Cider Vinegar And Detox

16. Apple Cider Vinegar And Dandruff

17. Apple Cider Vinegar And Gerd

18. Apple Cider Vinegar And Hair Loss

19. Apple Cider Vinegar And Constipation

20. Apple Cider Vinegar And Diabetes

Apple cider vinegar is great for you. With its so many benefits, it's no wonder why a lot of people are talking about apple cider vinegar and what it can do for your health.

If you find the idea of drinking full tablespoons of apple cider vinegar too difficult, taking apple cider vinegar pills may be a good alternative for you.

REASONS TO ADD APPLE CIDER VINEGAR TO YOUR DIET

- Experts suggest drinking a tablespoon of apple cider vinegar mixed with water or juice every day. Here are the reasons why.

- This liquid, which contains acetic acid, has antibiotic properties, which you need when suffering from diarrhea caused by a bacterial infection.

- The pectin in apple cider vinegar can help control intestinal spasms and indigestion.

- Do you have a sore throat? Gargle infections and nasty germs away with a concoction of a quarter cup of warm water and a quarter cup of your special vinegar. The acid will kill the germs.

- Scientists believe, after completing studies on animals, that your newly discovered sour mixture is also capable of lowering cholesterol in humans. More tests are needed.

- Are you often plagued by a stuffy nose or nasal congestion? The potassium in raw apple cider vinegar can thin mucus.

- Acetic acid can suppress a person's food cravings, reduce water retention, and increase metabolism. Consuming fewer calories equal weight loss.

- Nobody wants dandruff. Mix a quarter cup of water and a quarter cup of this unique type of vinegar in a spray bottle. Spritz it on your scalp before washing your hair.

- Wrap a towel around your head for 15 minutes. This routine should be done at least twice a week. Your hair will also be shinier.

- Need a boost of energy? You now know what to drink to beat fatigue!

- Individuals with eczema problems can clear up their skin and prevent outbreaks by ingesting ACV diluted in water.

- Stop bothersome nighttime leg cramps through the potassium found in apple cider vinegar. Make your new home remedy a little sweeter by adding a teaspoon of honey.

ADVANTAGES OF APPLE CIDER VINEGAR

The acid in the vinegar has been successfully used over and over to aid numerous skin conditions including bacterial overgrowth, removing the heavy residues left behind from soaps and shampoos and even aiding in such things as reducing acne outbreaks.

It improves hair and skin helping it maintain a more youthful appearance and is a useful disinfectant.

So if you want younger looking skin, fewer acne outbreaks, shiny, beautiful hair you need to start using apple cider vinegar. If you don't want to suffer from Candida, vaginal yeast infections or jock itch then you need this natural cure.

By placing apple vinegar and a little salt in your bath water you will make the water more neutral, making it a more natural bath which is great for skin and body odor. It is useful to bring apple cider vinegar on trips abroad when there are possible problems with contaminated food and water. Putting vinegar in water kills many types of bacteria and was used in ancient times for this very purpose.

In the same way when you drink a couple of teaspoons full of apple vinegar in 8oz`s of water just before a meal it can help kill food bound bacteria helping reduce the chance of food poisoning.

ADVANTAGES

1.   Bleeding: For hundreds of years, physicians have used vinegar for the treatment of wounds and to stop excess bleeding. For cuts and nosebleeds, you should soak a cotton ball in the vinegar and

place on the cut or place in the bleeding nose. It is also recommended by many to take internally before and after surgery.

2.   Allergies: It is believed that apple vinegar when taking as a daily tonic can boost immune function and improve metabolism which will aid in reducing many kinds of allergic reactions. Since asthma and arthritis are seen by some as an allergic reaction, it is often recommended for those conditions as well.

3.   Bone Health: Apple vinegar contains the minerals magnesium and manganese which improve health. It also contains the trace mineral boron which helps the body metabolize calcium and magnesium which help make strong bones.

4.   Blood Pressure: Apple cider vinegar is a good source of potassium which balances sodium in the body helping lower blood pressure.

APPLE CIDER VINEGAR HOME REMEDY

Although you may need to take medications to help ease nighttime heartburn, did you know that there is a natural apple cider vinegar acid reflux remedy you can try to ease symptoms during the day? Apple cider vinegar (ACV) is a natural treatment that has been used to treat a variety of ailments for many years and is a popular choice for acid reflux sufferers.

Apple Cider Vinegar contains what is known as the "mother of vinegar" or simply the "mother". The mother looks like stringy floating globs in the liquid and is where all of the healing properties of apple cider vinegar reside.

Apple cider vinegar contains minerals, as well as trace elements including magnesium, chlorine phosphorous, sulfur, sodium, calcium, potassium, iron, copper, fluorine and silicon.

Due of all of its beneficial ingredients, apple cider vinegar is a natural fighter of bacteria, which often makes it a beneficial vinegar acid reflux treatment choice.

How can apple cider vinegar benefit acid reflux sufferers? You may be confused as to how a type of vinegar could be beneficial for treating acid reflux symptoms such as heartburn.

After all, doesn't vinegar have a high acid content? Wouldn't cider vinegar just exacerbate the problem? Surprisingly, for most acid reflux sufferers, apple cider vinegar helps to relieve the burning sensation and nausea caused by reflux without adding to it.

Why? The reason is that many people with digestive problems like acid reflux, experience problems not because they have too much acid, but because they have too little.

Apple cider vinegar mimics the acid level of the stomach, which aids in the proper digestion of food, and can help aid the stomach in digesting.

Therefore, in some cases, vinegar acid reflux remedies for heartburn work more effectively than antacids, because although antacids will cure heartburn, they are designed to diminish acid within the system.

Thus, antacids will not treat the actual cause if acid reflux is the result of too little stomach acid, and instead can make reflux more frequent.

How should you take apple cider vinegar? Apple cider vinegar is available in many forms including liquid, tablet, and capsule.

However, when using apple cider vinegar as a natural treatment, the only form you should obtain is the organic liquid that contains the "mother" enzyme.

When taking apple cider vinegar, you will first want to shake it well before you ingest it to disperse the mother throughout the liquid. To start, try taking one tablespoon of cider vinegar before each meal.

You will likely find the taste of the apple cider vinegar to be quite potent. It is an acquired taste, and you should grow more accustomed to the flavor after the first few vinegar acid reflux treatments.

- Nevertheless, should you find it too repellant, there are a few other ways you can take apple cider vinegar such as?

- Mix a tablespoon in a fat-free salad dressing or light mayonnaise and eat it with your meal

- Sprinkle a tablespoon on salad or vegetables

- Mix a tablespoon in an 8 oz. glass of water and add a bit of honey to sweeten the drink.

- Make a tea out of apple cider vinegar by adding a tablespoon of the cider vinegar to hot water and slowly sipping it.

- Although it is best to ingest apple cider vinegar prior to each meal, you can also take a tablespoon when your stomach is upset or heartburn acts up.

After taking apple cider vinegar for a few days, many acid reflux sufferers find that their symptoms improve, and continue to improve with treatment in the months that follow.

However, in addition, you should be aware that Apple cider vinegar has a few mild side effects including stomach upset. Furthermore, Apple cider vinegar may worsen heartburn in some individuals.

It is also known to thin the blood and should be avoided by anyone taking blood thinning medications such as anticoagulants.

Always remember that you should speak to your doctor first before starting any treatment, including vinegar acid reflux treatment, and keep in mind that natural treatment should not replace any medication or treatment advice that has been prescribed by your doctor without prior consultation.

CHAPTER 4

HEALTH BENEFITS APPLE CIDER VINEGAR

When you think of apple cider, you probably think of fall. A warm sweet glass full of apples and spice that warms the body on a cool fall day and this delicious drink is where this miracle tonic gets its start.

It begins life as apples that are pulverized to make cider. This cider is then combined with yeast which turns the sugars in the cider into alcohol. From this point, the cider wine continues to ferment until it sours and turns into vinegar.

Apple cider vinegar has many claims to fame including:

- A natural acne fighter and skin toner

- A wart remover

- A hair rinse to brighten and nourish dull hair

- Removes lice, fleas, ticks, etc

- Cures infections

- Removes toxins

- A natural aftershave

- Relieves sunburn

And so much more!

The most important benefits of using apple cider vinegar are the effects that take place inside of the body. When added to your daily diet, its effects are pretty amazing. Let's take a look at a few of these benefits:

1. IMPROVED DIGESTION AND WEIGHT LOSS

Apple cider vinegar can help restore normal acid levels in your digestive system which helps break down fats and proteins. This allows your body to digest food easier and more thoroughly which promotes nutrient absorption by the body and overall health.

Apple cider vinegar can also help you feel fuller which will help you eat less and take some of the strain off of your digestive system. It is also been shown to help regulate blood sugar levels which promote weight loss and lowers the risk of diabetes.

One study also showed that regular supplementation with apple cider vinegar reduced body fat, triglyceride levels, and was effective for overall weight loss. It is a great weight loss supplement and an easy way to fight obesity.

2. HELPS PREVENT CANCER

Apple cider vinegar slows the growth of cancer cells and possibly even kills cancer cells. The results of studies have been somewhat contradictory on this subject but many possibilities are mentioned. Some think that the acetic acid in vinegar could be the cancer-fighting ingredient.

Others have proposed the pectin found in apples as well as polyphenols as possible anti-cancer ingredients. The true source is still a mystery but preliminary evidence has shown that apple cider vinegar is useful in the prevention of some forms of cancer.

3. IMPROVED CHOLESTEROL LEVELS AND BLOOD PRESSURE

A preliminary study performed in rats has shown that apple cider vinegar can significantly reduce cholesterol in the body. Since the study was performed on rats, some speculate that these properties may not be the same in humans. Further studies are needed to confirm but preliminary evidence is positive.

A similar study also showed positive results for lowering of blood pressure and heart disease as well. Due to the low number of side effects and the evidence suggesting it may reduce overall risk factors for heart disease, a regular dose of apple cider vinegar might be good advice.

4. LIVER AND OTHER ORGAN DETOXIFICATION

The anti-bacterial properties of apple cider vinegar help cleanse the body of toxic build-up as well as reduce levels of harmful bacteria. The body's PH balance is also stabilized by regular doses as well which helps to promote the natural cleansing effect of the body.

Apple cider vinegar has also been used to treat allergies as well by cleansing mucous out of the sinuses and cleansing the lymph nodes.

NOTE: When considering taking apple cider vinegar, make sure to find organic, unfiltered, and unpasteurized vinegar. You want untreated vinegar to maximize the health properties.

Before beginning any supplement program, even a natural one, speak with your doctor about possible side effects and interactions with any medications you are taking.

Apple cider vinegar can be taken straight from the bottle or through other forms such as pills to avoid the sour taste and acidity.

THE MIRACLE OF APPLE CIDER VINEGAR

Ever wonder what miracle cures lie in your home for various ailments? Next time you are in the grocery store, consider purchasing a bottle of apple cider vinegar.

You may just be surprised at how versatile and beneficial this inexpensive vinegar is. Apple cider vinegar contains various vitamins and minerals and has many health benefits.

Since before the dawn of our calendar, it has been reported that Hippocrates, the "father of medicine" used it for his patients. Apple cider vinegar is made from the fermentation of fresh, ripened apples. It contains such vitamins as beta-carotene and pectin, and such minerals as calcium, magnesium, phosphorus, potassium, and iron.

It can be used as a part of many recipes including salad dressings, marinades, meat tenderizers, and pickling. When searching for the best apple cider vinegar, look for natural and organic varieties that are dark and cloudy, as the sparkling clear types have very little nutritional value.

It can be consumed each morning, by adding two tablespoons to an 8-12oz. a glass of water, with organic honey and lemon juice if its taste is too potent due to its acidity. Apple cider vinegar is loaded with health benefits, with a sample listed below:

a.   Reducing cholesterol and regulating blood pressure and blood sugar due to its pectin content. May help with diabetes.

b.   Fights bacterial, fungal, and yeast infections by adjusting the body's pH due to its malic and acetic acid content.

c.   Can relieve joint pain and help with gout by dissolving uric acid crystals, as well as aid in preventing kidney and bladder stones.

d.   Helps with hair loss, brittle fingernails, and teeth due to its potassium content.

e.   Helps with weight loss by breaking down fats.

f.   Helps with acne, bad breath, and body odor because of its acid content, breaking down odor causing bacteria and lowering pH. Gargle one tablespoon of apple cider vinegar with water for five to ten minutes.

g.   Removes foot odor by placing feet in a pan of water and 1/3 cup of apple cider vinegar for 15 minutes per week.

h.   Helps with diarrhea as its pectin content coats the lining of the colon. Drink two tablespoons with a large glass of water, three times a day.

i.   May help with age spots, due to its sulfur content.

j.   Treats Dandruff by destroying fungus on the scalp, and restoring its proper pH balance. Try applying a mixture of half water and half apple cider vinegar directly to the scalp, allowing drying to occur naturally.

k.   Provides sunburn relief. Dampen a cloth with apple cider vinegar and gently apply to sunburn. You can also put the affected body part in a bath of apple cider vinegar.

l.   Boosts your immune system because of the beta-carotene that it possesses

m.   Can help with sinusitis and a runny nose due to its potassium content

n.   Helps with sore throats. Gargle with a tablespoon of apple cider vinegar and eight ounces of warm water, with lemon.

o.   Can help with ear infections, by dabbling a diluted solution of apple cider vinegar and sweeping the inner ear.

Many people choose to drink a diluted solution of apple cider vinegar and water daily for health benefits. Side effects are next to none, but can cause teeth enamel breakdown if consumed too often in a non-diluted state.

Simply add water or a pinch of baking soda when consuming to avoid any deterioration of enamel. From boosting immunity to helping regulate blood sugar, apple cider vinegar is very versatile.

A study in 2004 by the American Diabetes Society entitled,

"Vinegar Improves Insulin Sensitivity to a High-Carbohydrate Meal in Subjects with Insulin Resistance or Type 2 Diabetes" found that Apple cider vinegar contains acetic acid, which can slow down carbohydrate digestion, therefore lowering blood glucose levels.

Apple cider vinegar is easy and safe to purchase and use, and can be used as a wonderful alternative to aid your health.

It continues to be one of the most popular and inexpensive alternative health remedy on the market today.

CHAPTER 5

APPLE CIDER VINEGAR HEALTH CLAIMS WITH SCIENTIFIC EVIDENCE

Recently Apple cider vinegar has been deemed a very helpful health elixir. What once used to be considered folk remedies using this is now backed by scientific research indicating its helpful effects.

The primary ingredient is acetic acid. Vinegar also have other acids, vitamins, mineral salts and amino acids. Vinegar is a product of the process of fermentation by which sugars in a food are broken down by bacteria in yeast.

In the second stage of fermentation, the alcohol ferments further and we get vinegar. Specifically, Apple cider vinegar comes from crushed apples.

Because of the widespread claims that it can promote health benefits, scientific evidence has been evaluated and has shown that this indeed is true.

Extensive research has been conducted on blood sugar levels and this for the case of diabetes. Apple cider vinegar may help lower glucose levels in the blood. By consuming 2 tablespoons of apple cider vinegar prior to bedtime, lower glucose levels were found in the morning by four to six percent.

A study conducted in 2006 showed that it could lower cholesterol levels. The study, however, was done with rats, so it is not determined as to whether this would be experienced by people the same way. Another study conducted in rats showed a link between consumption of vinegar and lowering high blood pressure.

A few laboratory studies have shown that apple cider vinegar can kill cancer cells or inhibit their growth. Studies done with humans have inconclusive results.

On one hand consuming vinegar is associated with decreasing the risk of esophageal cancer while it is associated with increasing the risk of bladder cancer.

This may be helpful for the conscious dieter. Studies have shown consuming vinegar promotes fullness and fend off hunger. Controlling appetite can be a life-saving technique for those who are obese or are approaching obesity.

Popular home remedies involving this is abundant. A particular remedy for dandruff is to mix equal parts of apple cider vinegar and water. The vinegar solution restores the pH balance of the scalp and discourages the growth of the fungus which is the culprit causing dandruff.

When applied to acne, use one part vinegar to three parts water to make a vinegar solution. It is extremely important to dilute the vinegar so as not to damage the skin.

The popularity of Apple cider vinegar continues to this day. And the best part is that it is readily available at your local supermarket.

CHAPTER 6

APPLE CIDER VINEGAR IN TREATMENT OF CELLULITE

Cellulite is the fat deposited beneath the skin surface around the hips, buttocks, and thighs. Women of all races are afflicted by cellulite. It is seen mostly in obese women but does not exclusively spare lean women. Though cellulite per say is not indicative of any disease, it is often a cause of concern for cosmetic reasons.

The skin contains bands of elastic tissue that stretches from the skin to the deeper layers of the muscle tissue. These bands are inelastic and as fat is deposited in the subcutaneous area, the only way for it to move is to bulge out on the skin surface.

The strands of connective tissue try to keep the skin in place giving the dimpled effect to the skin. The formation of cellulite is mainly due to an imbalance in fatty acid metabolism. Other factors like lack of physical activity and improper diet are also responsible for cellulite deposition. Another contributory factor for cellulite formation is the poor circulation of blood and lymph which leads to accumulation of toxins in the body.

Many remedies are available for cellulite therapy and natural remedies are favored due to their safety profile.

Apple cider vinegar is one of the natural remedies used for the treatment of cellulite which has been known for over two thousand years in weight loss therapies.

Role of apple cider vinegar in cellulite therapy

1.   Apple cider vinegar strengthens the immune system and cures many infections. It also increases the body's metabolic rate and promotes thermogenesis.

2.   Due to the increased basal metabolic rate there is increased burning of fat which in turn balances cholesterol and causes weight loss.

3.   Other micronutrients present in apple cider vinegar like vitamin B6 and lecithin also contribute to weight loss. Since weight control is an essential aspect of cellulite therapy apple cider vinegar becomes extremely useful.

4.   Apple cider vinegar also helps in getting rid of the excess of fluids accumulated in the body by helping improve the circulation of blood.

5.   It is also known to curb the appetite.

6.   Apple cider vinegar is available for use as capsules or liquid. The capsules can be taken as two per day and can be increased to three doses a day if required. The liquid form can be used as two spoonfuls in a glass of water to be taken before every meal.

The advantages of apple cider vinegar is that it is a natural remedy with proven efficacy from ancient times in reducing weight apart from the fact that it is easy to use and effective.

CHAPTER 7

APPLE CIDER VINEGAR BEAUTY BENEFITS

Apple cider vinegar has become very popular because of its many health benefits and beauty properties. Because of its high potassium content, it is best to consult with a health care professional before taking Apple Cider Vinegar.

Although you can make your own apple cider vinegar, you can find it in a natural state at any health food store. Let's explore some of the benefits of apple cider vinegar.

HOW TO USE APPLE CIDER VINEGAR?

Apple cider vinegar can promote healthier skin and hair as well as be beneficial for health. For more specific ways in which apple cider can help treat specific ailments, contact a nutritionist who will be better equipped to answer specific questions. For more general uses, you can try apple cider vinegar in some of the following ways.

1.   INTERNAL USE

Research has shown that Apple Cider Vinegar can assist the body in its daily functions as well as fight off colds and influenza. It helps in digestion, lowers bad cholesterol, strengthens the heart, lowers blood pressure and stabilizes blood sugar. It also contains anti-oxidants that help fight some types of cancer.

It can cure an upset stomach by drinking it as a daily tonic.

To make your own daily tonic, mix equal parts of apple cider vinegar and honey in a glass of water.

Usually, one tablespoon of Apple Cider Vinegar and one tablespoon of honey in 8 ounces of warm or cold water would be a general guideline, but feel free to tweak this recipe depending on your personal preferences. There are also other ways to drink it.

You could add it to apple juice or add a bit of fresh cinnamon to neutralize its taste (some coffee shops serve apple cider with a cinnamon stick).

2.   EXTERNAL USE

If your feet feel tired and ache, give them a bath. Put half a cup of apple cider vinegar in a tub of warm water. Wiggle your toes around and let your feet soak for a few minutes. A footbath is a great way to relax before heading off to bed.

If your body is too acidic, take a vinegar bath. To properly restore the acid to alkaline balance in your body, simply add 1 to 2 cups of apple cider vinegar to a warm bath.

Soak your body for about 45 minutes. Aside from clearing your body from excess acid, a vinegar bath helps anyone with a dry or irritated skin making it feel soft.

If baths aren't your thing, consider mixing one cup each of Apple Cider Vinegar and warm water in a spray bottle. After your shower, spray your entire body with the mixture.

Wait a few minutes and rinse. Your whole body will feel refreshed.

Other benefits of apple cider vinegar include it's typically use on different body parts, especially the face. For a deep cleansing steam face wash, add 3 tablespoons of Apple Cider Vinegar to a pan of boiled water and lean your face over it. Cover your head with a towel for a few minutes to allow the steam to open up your pores and loosen any impurities from your skin's surface.

3.   COMMERCIAL PRODUCTS ON THE MARKET

Aside from the natural form of apple cider vinegar, many commercial products also exist. Such products include body washes and hair and facial products.

Taking Apple Cider Vinegar in its natural state is just as beneficial if not better than these products.

NOTE

Because Apple cider vinegar is very acidic, never drink it straight. Always dilute it with water. After drinking Apple Cider Vinegar, you should rinse your mouth with water. Also, do not brush your teeth right away because it might grind the vinegar into your enamel.

A great way to avoid Apple Cider Vinegar touching your teeth is to drink it with a straw. Apple Cider Vinegar tablets are a great alternative to the liquid, although they don't work as fast. Also, avoid eye contact with apple cider vinegar as the acid will burn and redden the eyes

The benefits of apple cider vinegar seem endless. These simple methods and ways of using Apple Cider Vinegar are all great and inexpensive. More importantly, they have proven methods beneficial to your body and to the environment. As long as you use it carefully and for recognized, healthy purposes, apple cider vinegar benefits will continue to reveal themselves. Try it for yourself.

CHAPTER 8

APPLE CIDER VINEGAR FOR BACTERIAL VAGINOSIS

Apple cider vinegar bacterial vaginosis treatment methods have been around for hundreds of years. After all, it is a natural substance. So, it has been around since long before modern medications were even invented.

One of the reasons that Apple cider vinegar has stuck around for so long is that it has many uses. It has antibacterial and mildly acidic properties, for example.

So, that makes it a good natural remedy for many illnesses, including Bacterial Vaginosis. Those same properties make this vinegar a great all natural cleaning product. Not only that, but it can even be an ingredient in many cooking recipes.

A NATURAL WAY TO TREAT BACTERIAL VAGINOSIS

Another reason that Apple cider vinegar has stayed so popular is that it is a natural way to treat Bacterial Vaginosis. It is slightly acidic, which can help to restore the pH levels within your body.

However, it isn't acidic enough to be harmful. Also, antibiotic treatments tend to only reduce Bacterial Vaginosis symptoms for a short time, not permanently. In fact, in general, natural cures and herbal remedies are much more apt to be supportive of your body than man-made chemical products are.

THE THREE APPLE CIDER VINEGAR APPLICATION METHODS

There are a lot of ways that you can treat or prevent bacterial vaginosis using apple cider vinegar. The best way to use it to prevent Bacterial Vaginosis is to drink just a little of it diluted in water each day.

However, you shouldn't drink more than a teaspoon in a large glass of water two times a day. In fact, once a day is probably enough.

Of course, you could also choose to douche with this vinegar, which is a good way to help cure an existing case of Bacterial Vaginosis. Two cups of water and a teaspoon of apple cider vinegar ought to do it.

However, you should only douche that way once per day. Over-douching can lead to a loss of good vaginal bacteria, as well as bad. So, it's important not to douche more than is absolutely necessary.

The third option is that you can simply bath in apple cider vinegar, but not in a full tub of it. You only need to use about one-half to one whole cup of it mixed into a shallow bath.

If you use too much vinegar, you will feel a severe burning sensation in your vaginal region. Also, you'll be likely to kill off all of the good bacteria in your vagina, which is never a good idea.

CHAPTER 9

GET RID OF HEARTBURN WITH APPLE CIDER VINEGAR

Apple cider vinegar is a folk remedy for getting rid of heartburn. In fact, it is the top folk remedy for heartburn and acid reflux.

RECIPE FOR RELIEF

Taking apple cider vinegar for heartburn relief is quite simple. Simply stir 2 Tablespoons of apple cider vinegar into 1/2 cup of water or apple juice. Drink this immediately after each meal.

If your problem is acid reflux, and you have just had a heavy meal, increase the amount of apple cider vinegar and decrease the amount of water or juice.

Another option is to mix a "cocktail" of the following:

- 1-quart apple juice

- 1-pint purple grape juice

- 1/2 cup apple cider vinegar

- Drink 1/2 cup after every meal for heartburn relief

Recipes that use apple cider vinegar for getting rid of heartburn vary greatly. This is because individual bodies also vary greatly. Try different amounts of apple cider vinegar until you find what works for you.

Some people have found that one brand or another works better for them. Again, the difference is due to the variations in physical makeup.

HOW APPLE CIDER VINEGAR REMEDIES HEARTBURN?

Little research has been done on the effectiveness of apple cider vinegar for heartburn relief. Consequently, it is difficult to say how apple cider vinegar remedies heartburn.

It appears that the acid content in vinegar somehow tells the stomach to stop producing more acid. Perhaps, in that way, apple cider vinegar is like the prescription medications that "shut down" the stomach's acid pumps to stop heartburn.

APPLES MAY HELP AS MUCH AS APPLE CIDER VINEGAR

Apple cider vinegar does not taste good to most people. Because of that, some have tried eating a few slices of apple after a meal, and have gotten rid of heartburn that way. Not every apple works for heartburn, though. Some stick to green apples such as Granny Smith.

Others recommend Jonagold apples for heartburn relief. Some recommend eating a few slices of Jonagold apple with a couple of dill pickle spears. It's apple cider vinegar for heartburn without resorting to basic vinegar.

NOTE: If you can get over the taste of apple cider vinegar, you will find it one of the most important natural remedies in healing the body.

CHAPTER 10

HOW TO USE ACV TO CURE ACNE?

If you want to try this vinegar acne treatment you have two options. The benefits refer to taking it internally (drinking it), but you can also use it externally.

Only apple cider vinegar is recommended for topical use. White vinegar and other forms of vinegar are often too strong.

Recipe for apple cider vinegar tonic:

- 2 tablespoons of apple cider vinegar

- 1/4 teaspoon of baking soda

- 1 cup of water

Just mix everything and drink it. Baking soda helps to neutralize acidity, which can cause dental problems. Skip the baking soda if you use this as a digestive aid.

In internal use, organic and unfiltered ACV (e.g. Braggs) gives the best results.

VINEGAR ACNE SCAR TREATMENT RECIPE

This recipe is particularly effective on acne scars, but it can also help to control pimples.

- Vinegar

- Water

Vinegar is an acid and it can feel like it's burning your skin. That's why it's recommended to dilute it with water. How much water you need depends on how sensitive your skin is.

Some people mix 50/50 water and vinegar, others mix 1 part vinegar with 3 parts water. Start with a weaker mixture and see how your skin reacts.

Vinegar for Acne scars is most often used as a toner. Apply it on your face, let it sit for few minutes and then wash off.

As you probably know, vinegar smells. So don't leave it on your skin if you plan to meet other people.

This recipe is rated as highly effective in a popular acne forum. Based on 363 votes, it has an overall rating of 4.3 out of 5 with 91% of the reviewers saying they would recommend it to others.

All said and done, Apple cider vinegar is unlikely to permanently cure acne. Aside from possibly helping with blood sugar control, it doesn't address the root cause of acne.

However, it's cheap and can be used to complement more effective acne treatment methods.

CHAPTER 10

HOW TO USE ACV TO CURE ACNE?

1. APPLE CIDER VINEGAR A NATURAL FAT BURNER.

Discover the incredible weight loss benefits of apple cider vinegar, how to best prepare it and how much you should use to get maximum benefit from apple cider vinegar - one of nature's amazing fat burning foods.

Here is the process: Apple juice is fermented to become alcohol containing apple cider. After that, oxygen is allowed to interact with the cider. This turns the alcohol into acetic acid. You will find this ingredient in the finished product.

What assists this process is spider-web-like foam of bacteria that is the result of the fermentation process. This is referred to as the "mother".

You can buy commercially prepared apple cider vinegar any time of year at specialty stores, health food stores, grocery stores, and supermarkets.

THE FAT FIGHTING BENEFITS OF APPLE CIDER VINEGAR

You can't beat this as a weapon in your battle with fat. There is no argument here. Actually, scientists have found that there are ninety different substances contained in it. Included are: 8 ethyl acetates, 18 kinds of alcohol, 20 types of ketones, 4 aldehydes, 13 kinds of carbolic acid, and more.

Here are some of the other great things you will find in it: Fiber in the form of potash and apple pectin, enzymes, amino, lactic, propionic and acetic acids, trace elements, minerals, and vitamins.

When we speak of health and fat fighting benefits, how does this information fit in? The following are the main benefits:

- The metabolism is sped up when apple cider vinegar is introduced. When you consume it before meals, this is even truer.

- It helps to process proteins and fats.

- It also helps increase metabolism and supports good digestive processes.

- It is low in fat, sugar, and salt.

It assists with the metabolism of minerals and fats. It aids in the digestion of greasy and fatty foods. It supports the liver in detoxifying the body. The body will burn calories better with the introduction of this vinegar. These are very beneficial in burning fat.

As a purifying and detoxifying agent, this particular vinegar is quite powerful. It helps to break down deposits of phlegm, mucous, and fat throughout the body.

Both your overall health and the functioning of your liver, bladder, kidneys and other areas of your body are assisted by this purifying and detoxifying process.

The reason for this is that it thins and oxidizes the blood and prevents an excess of alkaline in the urine. It helps prevent high blood pressure by thinning the blood.

This detoxification and purification can help to prevent the formation of harmful bacteria. It is also helpful in preventing inflammation and infections. Reduction of nasal discharge and the soothing of a sore throat can be accomplished with apple cider vinegar.

It detoxifies and purifies due to the potassium it contains. Poor health and toxic buildup may be the result of a lack of some salts and minerals. When this buildup occurs, the result can be boils, acne, blisters, and a variety of other symptoms.

It also assists in cleansing these buildups from the body. It also oxidizes the blood and supports healthy blood clotting.

The heart is benefited by the addition of potassium, which works to lower cholesterol and regulate blood pressure. Additionally, this is needed to help the body replace tissues that are worn.

Just as calcium helps repair bones, this ingredient helps with soft tissue repair. Hair loss can be prevented by the addition of potassium to the diet.

You will feel more energetic and vitality when you take this vinegar, thanks to the potassium and enzymes it includes.

Food is effectively broken down and digestion assisted thanks to hydrochloric acid and pepsin. This is an enzyme that is working within an acid environment. It assists in preventing indigestion.

Here are the benefits you will reap from the tartaric and malic acids found in this vinegar:

1.   Balanced acid levels.

2.   Eradication of negative bacteria found in the digestive tract.

This particular vinegar protects the immune system with its anti-fungal and antibacterial properties. It helps the blood to have a balanced alkalinity. This is because its high potassium electrolyte content assists in re-mineralizing the body.

Doctors and scientist think that it can help with symptoms of osteoporosis and arthritis. The reason for this is that it dissolves deposits of calcium around the joints and helps to strengthen bones.

The reason for this is the calcium, silicon, manganese, and magnesium content of the vinegar.

It has amino acids that work as antibiotics and antiseptics.

Toxicity in the body is reduced by the acetic acid found in this vinegar. It forms acetate compounds that assist in this process.

It helps to fight free radicals in the body because it is a powerful antioxidant. Free radicals are the harbingers of diseases such as heart disease and some forms of cancer.

It has antioxidant properties that assist it in neutralizing the free radicals that oxidation forms within our bodies.

It contains a water-soluble fiber called pectin. It helps to soak up cholesterol and fat in the body and carry them out in waste. Cholesterol is lowered by the use of this particular vinegar.

The fiber content protects against both diarrhea and constipation. Diabetics can benefit from the use of it because its dietary fiber is helpful in controlling blood glucose levels.

Macular degeneration, cataracts, and other eye diseases respond well to the addition of antioxidants and beta carotene to the diet. The vinegar is rich in these.

PREPARING APPLE CIDER VINEGAR

It is most often used when preparing salad dressings, pickles, and vegetable dishes. You will also find it in ketchup, mayonnaise, and mustard. You can use it as a condiment on veggie chips.

Chutneys and marinades benefit from the addition of a bit of it.

Additionally, you will note that you can substitute apple cider vinegar or lemon juice in a number of recipes.

This is especially so in some sorts of bread than in others. You may be worried that it will taste bitter, but it doesn't. Surprisingly, because of the apple content, it helps the dish to be very tasty.

It is fairly common knowledge that applesauce is a good substitute for oil or shortening when baking. Follow this principle and substitute it for lemon juice whenever it makes sense to do so. This gives you yet another alternative - happily, it is a healthy one.

Get started using this amazing vinegar with some of these ideas: When you begin to seek recipes actively, you will uncover quite a few?

Here are some of the dishes that benefit from the addition of apple cider vinegar:

- Baked goods

- Soups & stews

- Tandoori chicken

- Pickled goods

- Salad dressings

- Marinades & chutneys

- Sweet & sour chicken

- Caramelized onions

- Coleslaw

- Braised red cabbage

- Barbecued or baked tropical spareribs.

When you bake, you will not add apple cider vinegar to delicate baked goods. Nonetheless, bread is quite well suited for the addition it.

HOW MUCH APPLE CIDER VINEGAR SHOULD I USE?

Generally speaking, one tablespoon is the correct amount. This is the general amount for most recipes; however, be sure to read your recipe carefully. Whenever you add it to a drink, a tablespoon full is a good amount.

CONCLUSION

If you suffer from acid reflux, heartburn or nausea, try taking one tablespoon of Apple cider vinegar prior to each meal. You may see your symptoms go away in as little as three days.

However, you'll want to continue this practice for three to nine months and you may see the problem disappear altogether.

You don't want to use just any kind of Apple Cider vinegar, though. What you need is organic apple cider vinegar that still has the enzymes in it (called the "mother"). This is where the healing properties are.

The "mother" will show up inside the bottle as stringy globs floating around. To get the most out of your apple cider vinegar, shake it up each time you take a swig so that a mother can be dispersed throughout.

Certainly, most people do not take to the taste of Apple site of vinegar right away but it can be somewhat of an acquired taste and I know many people slug down a tablespoonful of the stuff all by itself.

If you can't stomach this, space, however, there are some things you can do to make it a little bit more palatable.

You might try making a tea from your Apple cider vinegar by heating a couple of water and then add a tablespoon of apple cider vinegar to that. You might also time to clean it with natural organic honey and some even say that this helps to boost the power.

While it's best to take apple cider vinegar before each meal, you can also take it anytime your stomach feels a little upset and it will have immediately curative effects.

Some people swear by it and drink it for everything including the onset of cold and flu. An additional benefit is that many people who have taken apple cider vinegar before each meal have seen a moderate weight loss as well.

You know what they say, an apple a day keeps the doctor away - well, in this case, it's a swig of apple cider vinegar today.